Healthy Keto Vegetarian Cookbook

Lose Weight and Feel Great with these Easy to Cook Plant-Based Keto Vegetarian Recipes

Lidia Wong

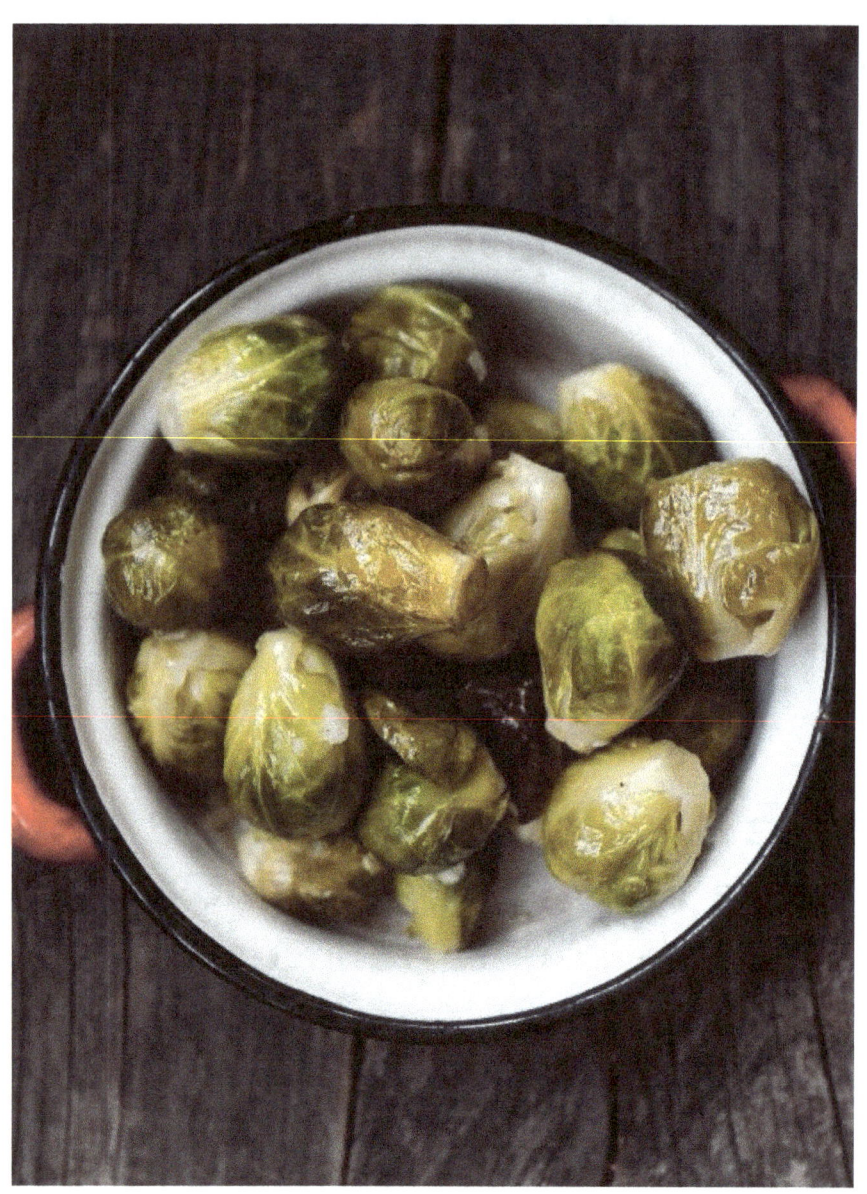

© **Copyright 2021 by Lidia Wong - All rights reserved.**

The content contained within this book may not be reproduced, duplicated or transmitted without direct written permission from the author or the publisher.
Under no circumstances will any blame or legal responsibility be held against the publisher, or author, for any damages, reparation, or monetary loss due to the information contained within this book. Either directly or indirectly.

Legal Notice:
This book is copyright protected. This book is only for personal use. You cannot amend, distribute, sell, use, quote or paraphrase any part, or the content within this book, without the consent of the author or publisher.

Disclaimer Notice:
Please note the information contained within this document is for educational and entertainment purposes only. All effort has been executed to present accurate, up to date, and reliable, complete information. No warranties of any kind are declared or implied. Readers acknowledge that the author is not engaging in the rendering of legal, financial, medical or professional advice. The content within this book has been derived from various sources. Please consult a licensed professional before attempting any techniques outlined in this book.
By reading this document, the reader agrees that under no circumstances is the author responsible for any losses, direct or indirect, which are incurred as a result of the use of information contained within this document, including, but not limited to, — errors, omissions, or inaccuracies.

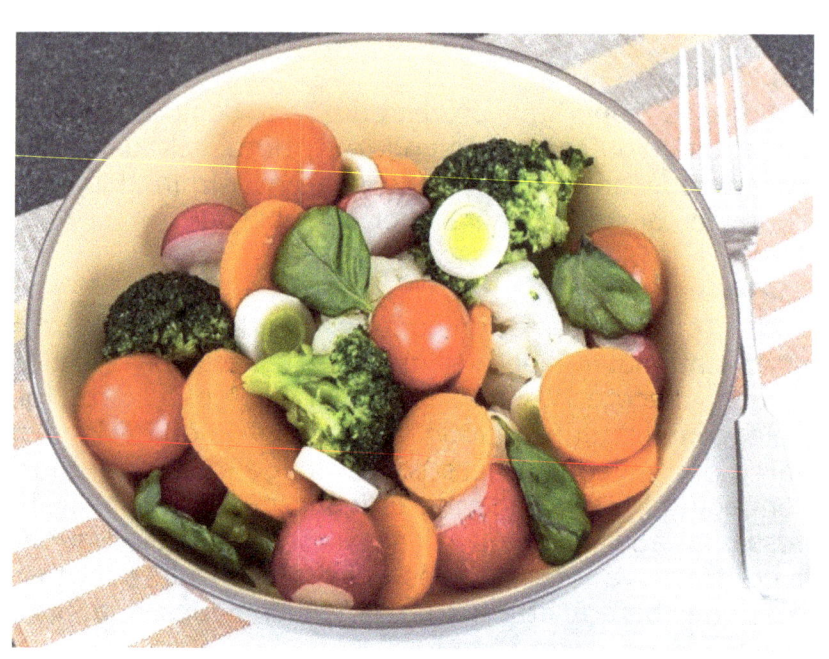

TABLE OF CONTENTS

INTRODUCTION 1

Roasted Peppers Muffins 3

Healthy Breakfast Porridge 5

Zucchini Muffins 6

Soy Chorizo, Eggs & Feta Cheese Plate 8

Cauliflower and Artichokes Soup 10

Hot Cabbage Soup 12

Hot Cranberries and Arugula Mix 14

Mushrooms and Asparagus Mix 15

Sage Rice and Veggies 17

Arugula Tomato Salad 19

Avocado Cilantro Dip 20

Vegan Sausage with Vegan Bacon 21

Chard and Peppers Mix 23

Spinach Mash 25

Tomato and Walnuts Vinaigrette 27

Turmeric Carrots 28

Beets And Carrots 29

Flavored Tomato and Okra Mix 30

- Wild Mushrooms and Radish Rice 32
- Grilled Portobello with Mashed Potatoes and Green Beans 34
- Eggplant Hash 38
- Eggplant Jam 40
- Artichokes and Tomatoes Dip 42
- Rhubarb and Strawberry Compote 44
- Roasted Tomato Cream 46
- Sweet Potato And Peanut Soup With Baby Spinach 48
- Zoodle Bolognese 50
- Keto Pasta with Mediterranean Tofu balls 53
- Spinach Salad With Orange-Dijon Dressing 57
- Warm Lentil Salad with Red Wine Vinaigrette 59
- Tabbouleh Salad 62
- Yellow Mung Bean Salad With Broccoli And Mango 64
- Baked Onion Rings 66
- Corn Cream Soup 68
- Corn And Cabbage Soup 70
- Okra Soup 72
- Baby Carrots And Coconut Soup 74
- Nut Free Nacho Dip (vegan) 76

Black Olive & Thyme Cheese Spread (vegan).......... 78

Curry with Bok Choy 80

Capers Dip... 82

Apple Crumble... 83

Peach-Mango Crumble (Pressure cooker)................. 86

Coconut and Almond Truffles 88

Avocado and Pineapple Bowls 90

Mint Cookies... 91

Sweet Zucchini Buns 93

Peppermint Patty Cocoa 95

Maple & Rum Apples. 96

Zucchini bread... 98

Fat-Rich Protein Espresso (vegan) 101

NOTE **103**

INTRODUCTION

The keto diet is the shortened term for ketogenic diet and it is essentially a high-fat and low-carb diet that helps you lose weight, thereby bringing various health benefits. This diet drastically restricts your carb intake while increasing your fat intake; this pushes your body to go into a state know as "*ketosis*". We will tackle ketosis in a bit.

The human body uses glucose from carbs to fuel metabolic pathways—meaning various bodily functions like digestion, breathing, etc.. Essentially, anything that needs energy. Even when you are resting, the body needs fuel or energy for you to continue living. If you think about it, when have you ever stopped breathing, or your heart stopped beating, or your liver stopped from cleansing the body, or your kidneys from filtering blood?

Never, unless you're dead, which is the only time in which the body doesn't need energy. In normal circumstances, glucose is the primary pathway when it comes to sourcing the body's energy.

But the body also has another pathway; it can utilize fats to fuel the various bodily processes. And this is what we call "*ketosis*". And the body can only enter ketosis when there is no glucose available, thus the reason for sticking to a low-carb diet is essential in the keto diet. Since no glucose is available, the body is pushed to use fats—it can either come from the food you consume or from your body's fat reserves—the adipose tissue or from the flabby parts of your body. This is how the keto diet helps you lose weight, by burning up all those stored fats that you have and using it to fuel bodily processes.

That said, if for whatever reason you are a vegetarian, following a ketogenic diet can be extremely difficult. A vegetarian diet is largely free of animal products, which means that food tends to be usually high in carbohydrates. Still, with careful planning, it is possible. This Cookbook will provide you with various easy and delicious dishes to help you stick to your ketogenic diet plan while being a vegetarian.

Enjoy!

Roasted Peppers Muffins

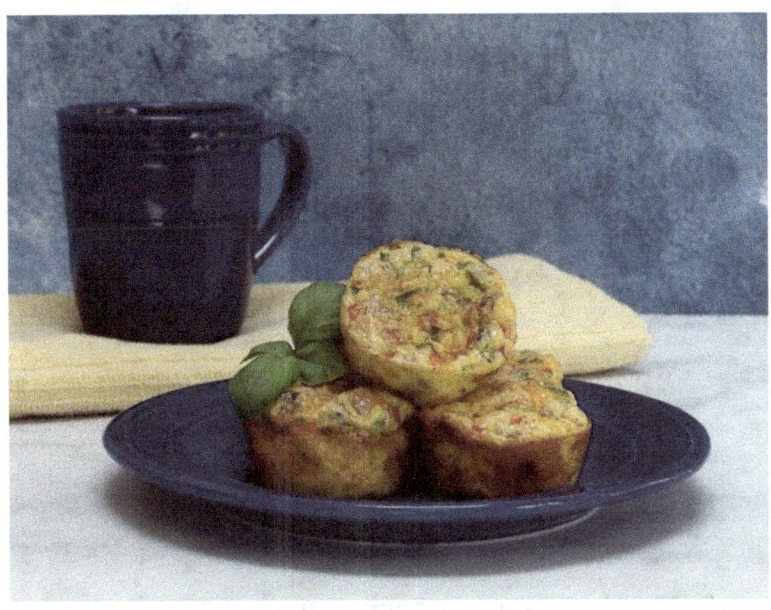

Preparation time: 10 minutes

Cooking time: 15 minutes

Servings: 6

Ingredients:

- 2 tablespoons flaxseed mixed with 3 tablespoons water
- ½ cup coconut cream
- 1/3 cup spinach, chopped

- ¼ cup cashew cheese, grated
- ½ cup roasted red peppers, chopped
- A pinch of salt and black pepper
- 2 tablespoons oregano, chopped
- 1 teaspoon chili powder
- Cooking spray

Directions:

1. In a bowl, combine the spinach with the flaxseed mix, the cream and the other ingredients except the cooking spray, and whisk well.
2. Grease a muffin pan with the cooking spray, divide the peppers mix, bake at 400 degrees F for 15 minutes and serve for breakfast.

Nutrition:

calories 209, fat 16.7, fiber 1.8, carbs 6.8, protein 9.3

Healthy Breakfast Porridge

Preparation Time: 5 minutes

Cooking Time: 5 minutes

Servings: 2

Ingredients:

- 4 tablespoons coconut, unsweetened, shredded
- 1 tablespoon oat bran
- 1/8 teaspoon salt
- 1 tablespoon flaxseed meal
- ½ tablespoon butter
- ¾ teaspoon Truvia
- ½ teaspoon cinnamon
- ½ cup heavy cream
- 1 cup water

Directions:

1. Add all your ingredients into a saucepan over medium-low heat. Once the mixture comes to a boil remove from heat. Serve warm and enjoy!

Nutritional Values (Per Serving):

Calories: 222 Fat: 21 g Carbohydrates: 3.90 g Sugar: 3.9 g Protein: 2.68 g, Cholesterol: 49 mg

Zucchini Muffins

Preparation Time: 10 minutes

Cooking Time: 35 minutes

Serving: 6

Ingredients:

- ½ cup almond flour
- 1 tsp baking powder
- 2 zucchinis, grated
- ½ tsp baking soda
- 1/3 cup almond milk
- 1 ½ tsp mustard powder
- Salt and black pepper to taste
- 1 large egg
- 5 tbsp olive oil
- ½ cup grated cheddar cheese
- 6 green olives, pitted and sliced
- 1 spring onion, finely chopped
- 1 small red bell pepper, deseeded and chopped
- 1 tbsp freshly chopped thyme

Directions:

1. Preheat the oven to 325 °F and grease a pan with cooking spray.
2. In a large bowl, combine the almond flour, baking powder, baking soda, mustard powder, salt, black pepper. In a smaller bowl, whisk the milk, egg, and olive oil. Mix the wet ingredients into the dry ingredients and add the cheese, zucchini, olives, spring onion, bell pepper, and thyme. Combine well.
3. Spoon the batter into the muffin holes, ¾-inch full and bake in the oven for 30 to 35 minutes or until golden brown on top and skewer inserted comes out clean.
4. Remove the pan from the oven and allow the muffins to cool in a tin for 10 minutes before removing.
5. Serve immediately for brunch.

Nutrition:

Calories:137, Total Fat: 9.5g, Saturated Fat:4.4 g, Total Carbs: 3 g, Dietary Fiber: 0g, Sugar:1 g, Protein: 1g, Sodium: 1001mg

Soy Chorizo, Eggs & Feta Cheese Plate

Preparation Time: 10 minutes

Cooking time: 5 minutes

Serving: 4

Ingredients:

- 4 eggs
- 1 tsp olive oil
- 1 tsp smoked paprika
- 3 oz soy chorizo, diced
- ½ cup crumbled feta cheese
- 2 green onions, thinly sliced diagonally
- 2 tbsp fresh parsley, chopped
- Greek yogurt to serve

Directions:

1. Preheat the oven to 350 °F.
2. On a stovetop over medium temperature, heat the olive oil along with the paprika in an oven safe non-stick frying pan for 30 seconds. Add the soy chorizo and cook until lightly browned; spoon the soy chorizo into a bowl, leaving the

olive oil in the pan.
3. Crack the eggs into the pan, cook for 2 minutes, and then sprinkle with the chorizo and crumble the feta cheese all around the egg white, but not on the yolks.
4. Transfer the pan to the oven and bake for 1 to 2 more minutes or until the yolks are quite set, but still runny within.
5. Remove the pan, garnish with the green onions and parsley.
6. Serve warm with Greek yogurt.

Nutrition:

Calories:414, Total Fat: 34.7g, Saturated Fat:19.3 g, Total Carbs: 2 g, Dietary Fiber:0 g, Sugar: 0g, Protein: 24g, Sodium: 639mg

Cauliflower and Artichokes Soup

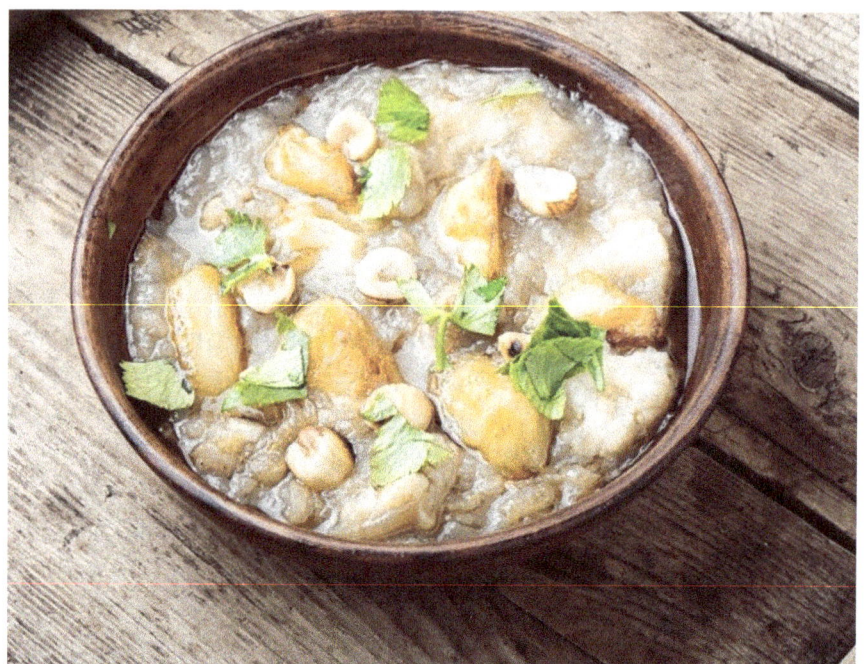

Preparation time: 10 minutes

Cooking time: 25 minutes

Servings: 4

Ingredients:

- 1 pound cauliflower florets
- 1 cup canned artichoke hearts, drained and chopped

- 2 garlic cloves, minced
- 2 scallions, chopped
- 2 tablespoons olive oil
- 6 cups vegetable stock
- Salt and black pepper to the taste
- 2/3 cup coconut cream
- 2 tablespoons cilantro, chopped

Directions:

1. Heat up a pot with the oil over medium heat, add the scallions and the garlic and sauté for 5 minutes.
2. Add the cauliflower and the other ingredients, toss, bring to a simmer and cook over medium heat for 20 minutes more.
3. Blend the soup using an immersion blender, divide it into bowls and serve.

Nutrition:

calories 207, fat 17.2, fiber 6.2, carbs 14.1, protein 4.7

Hot Cabbage Soup

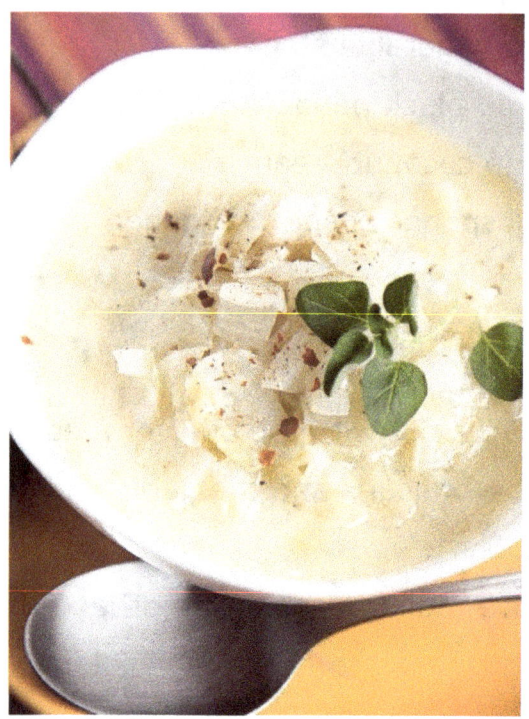

Preparation time: 10 minutes

Cooking time: 30 minutes

Servings: 4

Ingredients:

- 1 green cabbage head, shredded
- 3 spring onions, chopped

- 6 cups vegetable stock
- 2 tablespoons olive oil
- 1 tablespoon ginger, grated
- 1 teaspoon cumin, ground
- Salt and black pepper to the taste
- 1 teaspoon hot paprika
- 1 teaspoon chili powder
- 1 tablespoon cilantro, chopped

Directions:

1. Heat up a pot with the oil over medium heat, add the spring onions, ginger and the cumin and sauté for 5 minutes.
2. Add the cabbage and the other ingredients, stir, bring to a simmer and cook over medium heat for 25 minutes more.
3. Ladle the soup into bowls and serve for lunch.

Nutrition:

calories 117, fat 7.5, fiber 5.2, carbs 12.7, protein 2.8

Hot Cranberries and Arugula Mix

Preparation time: 10 minutes

Cooking time: 0 minutes

Servings: 4

Ingredients:

- 1 cucumber, cubed
- 1 cup cranberries
- 2 cups baby arugula
- 1 avocado, peeled, pitted and cubed
- ¼ cup kalamata olives, pitted and sliced
- 1 tablespoon walnuts, chopped
- 2 tablespoons olive oil
- 2 tablespoons lime juice

Directions:

1. In a bowl, combine the arugula with the cranberries and the other ingredients, toss well, divide between plates and serve.

Nutrition:

calories 110, fat 4, fiber 2, carbs 10, protein 2

Mushrooms and Asparagus Mix

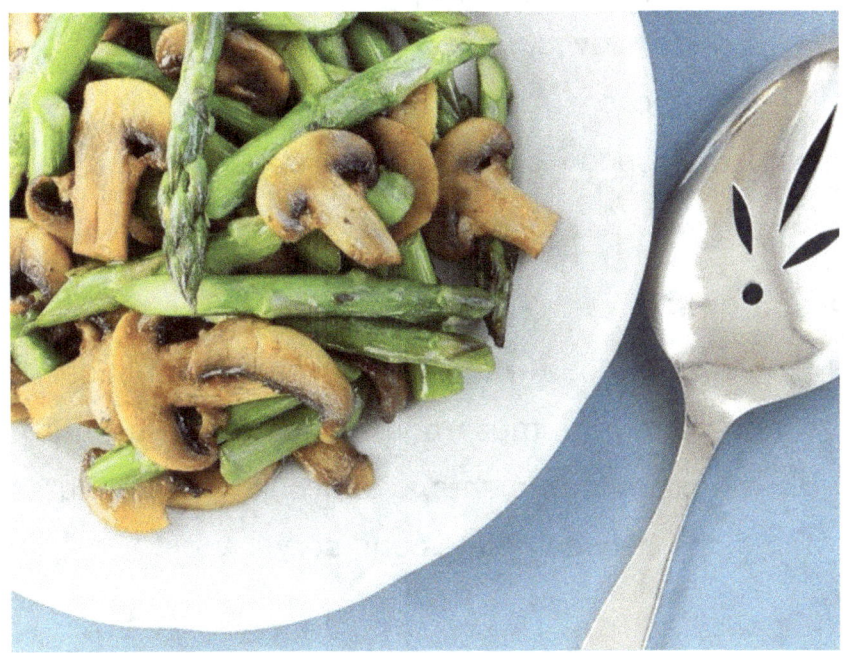

Preparation time: 10 minutes

Cooking time: 15 minutes

Servings: 4

Ingredients:

- 1 pound white mushrooms, sliced
- 1 asparagus bunch, trimmed and halved
- 1 teaspoon sweet paprika

- 1 teaspoon coriander, ground
- 1 teaspoon chili powder
- ½ teaspoon thyme, dried
- 2 garlic cloves, minced
- ¼ cup coconut cream
- 1 tablespoon avocado oil

Directions:

1. Heat up a pan with the oil over medium high heat, add the mushrooms, the asparagus and the other ingredients, toss, cook for 15 minutes, divide between plates and serve.

Nutrition:

calories 74, fat 4.6, fiber 2.6, carbs 6.9, protein 4.7

Sage Rice and Veggies

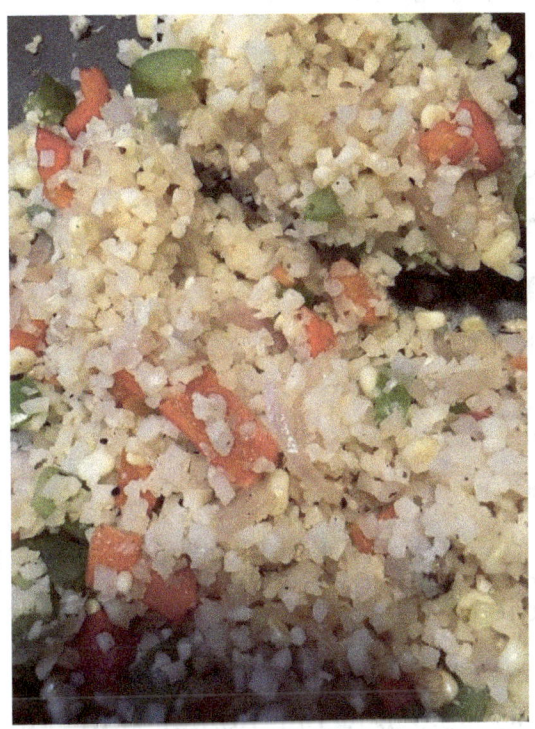

Preparation time: 10 minutes

Cooking time: 12 minutes

Servings: 4

Ingredients:

- 2 cups cauliflower rice
- 2 tablespoons olive oil

- 1 green bell pepper, chopped
- 1 avocado, peeled, pitted and cubed
- 1 green chili, chopped
- ½ cup radishes, halved
- 1 tomato, cubed
- 1 zucchini, cubed
- 1 tablespoon sage, chopped
- 1 teaspoon lime juice
- A pinch of salt and black pepper

Directions:

1. Heat up a pan with the oil over medium heat, add the green chili and the cauliflower rice and sauté for 2 minutes.
2. Add the avocado, bell pepper and the other ingredients, toss, cook over medium heat for 10 minutes more, divide between plates and serve.

Nutrition:

calories 202, fat 17.1, fiber 6.3, carbs 13.2, protein 3.2

Arugula Tomato Salad

Preparation Time: 20 minutes

Servings: 2

Ingredients:

- 4 tablespoons olive oil
- 1 small red onion, chopped
- 1 cup cherry tomatoes, halved
- 3 cups arugula, washed, drained
- 4 tablespoons capers, canned, drained
- 2 tablespoons basil, fresh, chopped

Directions:

1. Add all ingredients into mixing bowl and toss.
2. Serve fresh and enjoy!

Nutritional Values (Per Serving):

Calories: 262 Fat: 26.7 g Carbohydrates: 6 g Sugar: 3.1 g Protein: 2.1 g Cholesterol: 0 mg

Avocado Cilantro Dip

Preparation Time: 10 minutes

Servings: 2

Ingredients:

- 1 cup cilantro, fresh
- ½ teaspoon onion powder
- 1 garlic clove
- ½ cup sour cream
- 1 fresh lemon juice
- 2 avocados
- ¼ teaspoon sea salt

Directions:

1. Using your blender blend ingredients, and blend until smooth. Place the mixture in your fridge to combine flavors for a few hours.
2. Serve with crackers and enjoy!

Nutritional Values (Per Serving):

Calories: 273 Cholesterol: 13 mg Sugar: 2.1 g Fat: 25.7 g Carbohydrates: 11.6 g Protein: 3 g

Vegan Sausage with Vegan Bacon

Preparation Time: 5 minutes

Cooking Time: 40 minutes

Serving: 4

Ingredients:

- 8 large vegan sausages
- 1 tsp onion powder
- ½ cup grated Swiss cheese
- 16 slices vegan bacon
- 1 tsp garlic powder
- Salt and black pepper to taste

Directions:

1. Preheat the oven to 400 ^{0}F.
2. Cut a slit in the middle of each vegan sausage and stuff evenly with the Swiss cheese.
3. Wrap each vegan sausage with 2 vegan bacon slices each and secure with toothpicks.
4. Season with the onion powder, garlic powder, salt, and black pepper.

5. Place the wrapped vegan sausage on a baking sheet and place in the middle rack of the oven.
6. Cook for 35 to 40 minutes or until the bacon browns and crisps.
7. Remove the food and serve warm with your preferred side dish.

Nutrition:

Calories:639, Total Fat: 55.6g, Saturated Fat:4.6 g, Total Carbs: 9 g, Dietary Fiber: 2g, Sugar: 2g, Protein:28 g, Sodium: 999mg

Chard and Peppers Mix

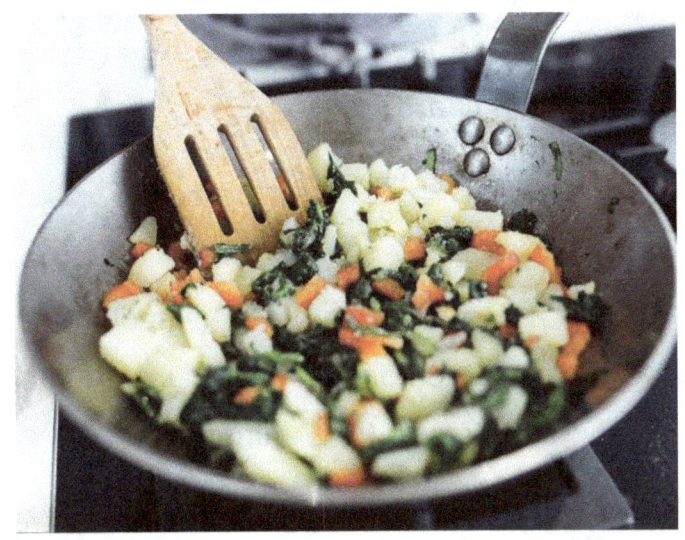

Preparation time: 10 minutes

Cooking time: 20 minutes

Servings: 4

Ingredients:

- 2 tablespoons avocado oil
- 2 spring onions, chopped
- 2 tablespoons capers, drained
- 2 tablespoons tomato passata
- 2 green bell peppers, cut into strips

- A pinch of cayenne pepper
- 1 teaspoon turmeric powder
- Juice of 1 lime
- Salt and black pepper to the taste
- 1 bunch red chard, torn

Directions:

1. Heat up a pan with the oil over medium heat, add the spring onions, capers, turmeric and cayenne and sauté for 5 minutes.
2. Add the peppers, chard and the other ingredients, toss, cook over medium heat for 15 minutes more, divide between plates and serve.

Nutrition:

calories 119, fat 7, fiber 3, carbs 7, protein 2

Spinach Mash

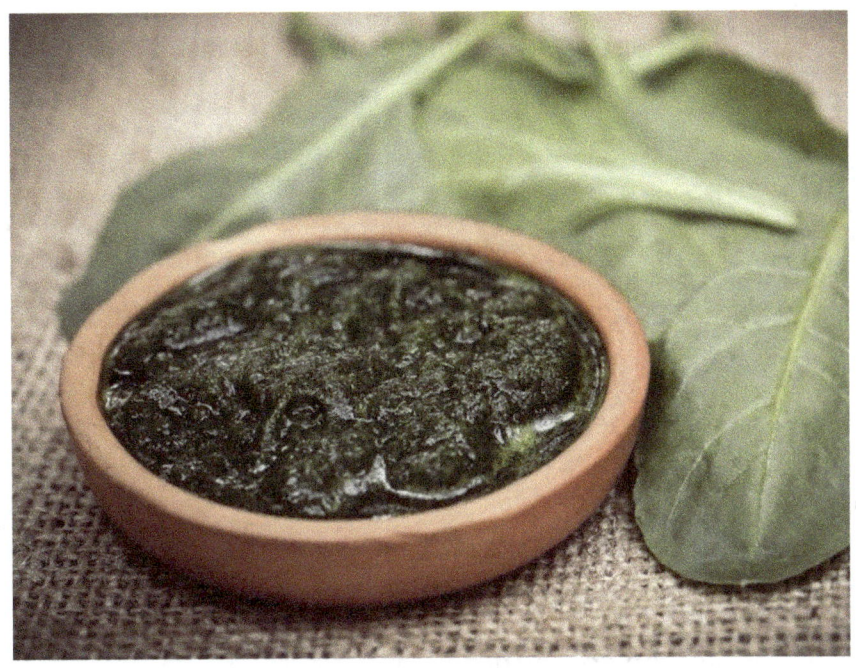

Preparation time: 10 minutes

Cooking time: 15 minutes

Servings: 4

Ingredients:

- 1 pound spinach leaves
- 2 garlic cloves, minced
- 3 scallions, chopped

- ¼ cup coconut cream
- 2 tablespoons olive oil
- Salt and black pepper to the taste
- ½ tablespoon chives, chopped

Directions:

1. Heat up a pan with the oil over medium heat, add the scallions and the garlic and sauté for 2 minutes.
2. Add the spinach and the other ingredients except the chives, toss, cook over medium heat for 13 minutes, blend using an immersion blender, divide between plates, sprinkle the chives on top and serve.

Nutrition:

calories 190, fat 16, fiber 7, carbs 3, protein 5

Tomato and Walnuts Vinaigrette

Preparation time: 10 minutes

Cooking time: 0 minutes

Serving: 4

Ingredients:

- 1 pound cherry tomatoes, halved
- 1 tablespoon walnuts, chopped
- 2 teaspoons smoked paprika
- 1 tablespoon balsamic vinegar
- 1 garlic clove, minced
- 1 teaspoon lemon juice
- ¼ teaspoon coriander, ground
- Salt and black pepper to the taste
- 1 tablespoon parsley, chopped

Directions:

1. In a bowl, combine the tomatoes with the walnuts and the other ingredients, toss well, and serve as a side dish.

Nutrition:

calories 160, fat 12, fiber 4, carbs 6, protein 4

Turmeric Carrots

Preparation time: 10 minutes

Cooking time: 40 minutes

Servings: 4

Ingredients:

- 1 pound baby carrots, peeled
- 1 tablespoon olive oil
- 1 teaspoon turmeric powder
- 1 tablespoon chives, chopped
- 2 spring onions, chopped
- 2 tablespoons balsamic vinegar
- 2 garlic cloves, minced
- ¼ teaspoon cayenne pepper
- A pinch of salt and black pepper

Directions:

1. Spread the carrots on a baking sheet lined with parchment paper, add the oil, the spring onions and the other ingredients, toss and bake at 380 degrees F for 40 minutes.
2. Divide the carrots between plates and serve.

Nutrition:

calories 79, fat 3.8, fiber 3.7, carbs 10.9, protein 1

Beets And Carrots

Preparation time: 10 minutes

Cooking time: 7 hours

Servings: 8

Ingredients:

- 2 tablespoons stevia
- 2 and ½ pounds beets, peeled and cut into wedges
- ¾ cup pomegranate juice
- 2 teaspoons ginger, grated
- 12 ounces carrots, cut into medium wedges

Directions:

1. In your slow cooker, mix beets with carrots, ginger, stevia and pomegranate juice, toss, cover and cook on Low for 7 hours.
2. Divide between plates and serve as a side dish.
3. Enjoy!

Nutrition:

calories 125, fat 0, fiber 4, carbs 28, protein 3

Flavored Tomato and Okra Mix

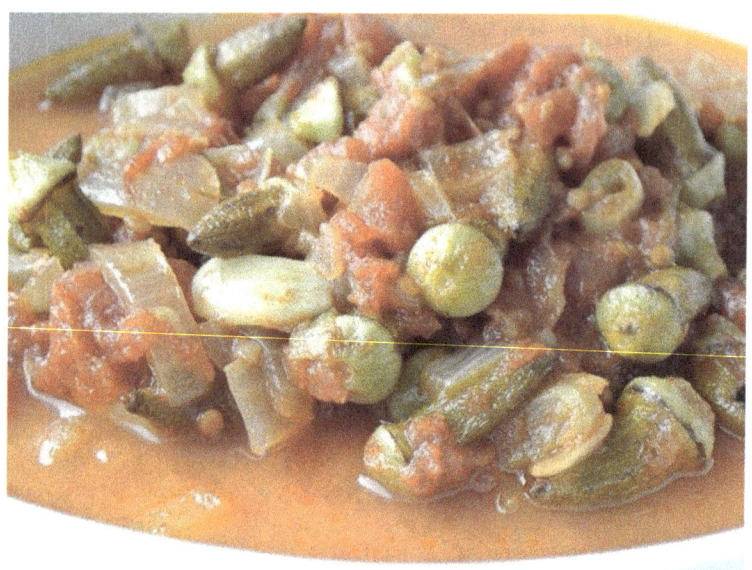

Preparation time: 10 minutes

Cooking time: 30 minutes

Servings: 6

Ingredients:

- 2 cups okra, sliced
- 1 cup scallions, chopped
- 1 pound cherry tomatoes, halved
- 2 tablespoons avocado oil

- 4 garlic cloves, chopped
- 2 teaspoons oregano, dried
- 2 teaspoons cumin, ground
- A pinch of salt and black pepper
- 1 cup veggie stock
- 2 tablespoons tomato passata

Directions:

1. Heat up a pan with the oil over medium heat, add the scallions and the garlic and sauté for 5 minutes.
2. Add the tomatoes, the okra and the other ingredients, toss, cook over medium heat for 25 minutes, divide between plates and serve as a side dish.

Nutrition:

calories 84, fat 2.1, fiber 5.4, carbs 14.8, protein 4

Wild Mushrooms and Radish Rice

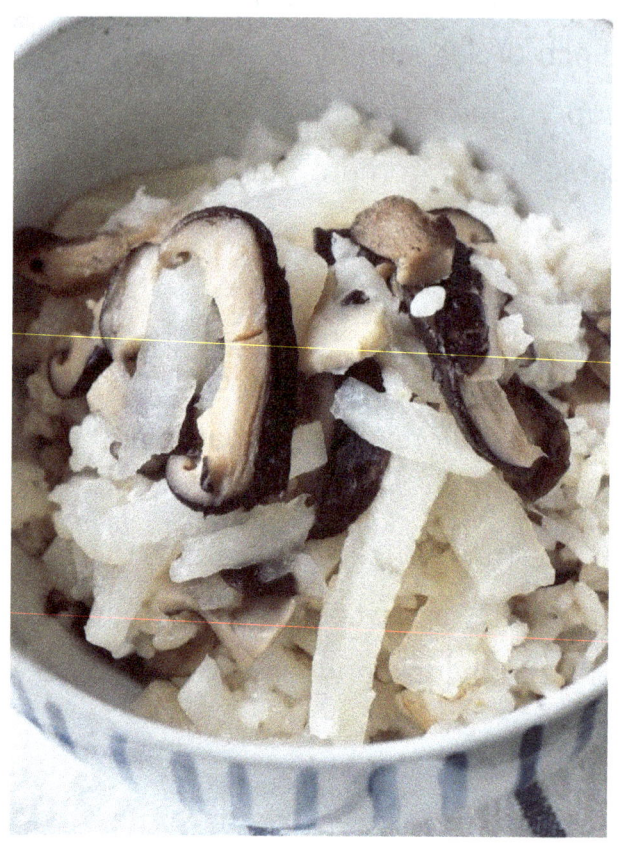

Preparation time: 10 minutes

Cooking time: 25 minutes

Servings: 4

Ingredients:

- 2 cups cauliflower rice
- ½ cup radishes, halved
- 3 shallots, chopped
- 2 tablespoons avocado oil
- ½ cup wild mushrooms, sliced
- 1 cup veggie stock
- 1 teaspoon fennel seeds
- 1 teaspoon coriander, ground
- A pinch of salt and black pepper
- 2 tablespoons chives, chopped

Directions:

1. Heat up a pan with the oil over medium heat, add the shallots and the mushrooms and sauté for 5 minutes.
2. Add the cauliflower rice, the radishes and the other ingredients, toss, cook over medium heat for 20 minutes, divide between plates and serve as a side dish.

Nutrition:

calories 189, fat 3, fiber 4, carbs 9, protein 8

Grilled Portobello with Mashed Potatoes and Green Beans

Preparation time: 20 minutes

cooking time: 40 minutes

servings: 4

Ingredients

For the grilled portobellos

- 4 large portobello mushrooms
- 1 teaspoon olive oil
- Pinch sea salt

For the mashed potatoes

- 3 to 4 garlic cloves, minced
- 6 large potatoes, scrubbed or peeled, and chopped
- ½ teaspoon olive oil
- ½ cup non-dairy milk
- 2 tablespoons coconut oil (optional
- 2 tablespoons nutritional yeast (optional)
- Pinch sea salt

For the green beans

- 2 cups green beans, cut into 1-inch pieces
- 2 to 3 teaspoons coconut oil
- Pinch sea salt
- 1 to 2 tablespoons nutritional yeast (optional)

Directions

To Make The Grilled Portobellos

1. Preheat the grill to medium, or the oven to 350 °F.
2. Take the stems out of the mushrooms.
3. Wipe the caps clean with a damp paper towel, then dry them. Spray the caps with a bit of olive oil, or put some oil in your hand and rub it over the mushrooms.
4. Rub the oil onto the top and bottom of each mushroom, then sprinkle them with a bit of salt on top and bottom.
5. Put them bottom side facing up on a baking sheet in the oven, or straight on the grill. They'll take about 30 minutes in the oven, or 20 minutes on the grill. Wait until they're soft and wrinkling around the edges.

6. If you keep them bottom up, all the delicious mushroom juice will pool in the cap. Then at the very end, you can flip them over to drain the juice.
7. If you like it, you can drizzle it over the mashed potatoes.

To Make The Mashed Potatoes

8. Boil the chopped potatoes in lightly salted water for about 20 minutes, until soft. While they're cooking, sauté the garlic in the olive oil, or bake them whole in a 350 °F oven for 10 minutes, then squeeze out the flesh.
9. Drain the potatoes, reserving about ½ cup water to mash them.
10. In a large bowl, mash the potatoes with a little bit of the reserved water, the cooked garlic, milk, coconut oil (if using), nutritional yeast (if using), and salt to taste.
11. Add more water, a little at a time, if needed, to get the texture you want. If you use an immersion blender or beater to purée them, you'll have some extra-creamy potatoes.

To Make The Green Bean

12. Heat a medium pot with a small amount of water to boil, then steam the green beans by either putting them directly in the pot or in a steaming basket.
13. Once they're slightly soft and vibrantly green, 7 to 8 minutes, take them off the heat and toss them with the oil, salt, and nutritional yeast (if using).

Nutrition:

Calories: 263; Total fat: 7g; Carbs: 43g; Fiber: 7g; Protein: 10g

Eggplant Hash

Preparation time: 20 minutes

Cooking time: 20 minutes

Servings: 4

Ingredients:

- 1 eggplant, roughly chopped
- ½ cup olive oil
- ½ pound cherry tomatoes, halved
- ¼ cup basil, chopped
- ¼ cup mint, chopped
- 1 teaspoon Tabasco sauce
- A pinch of sea salt
- Black pepper to taste

Directions:

1. Put eggplant pieces in a bowl, add a pinch of salt, toss to coat, leave aside for 20 minutes and drain using paper towels.
2. Heat up a pan with half of the oil over medium-high heat, add eggplant, cook for 3 minutes, flip, cook them for 3 minutes more and transfer

to a bowl.
3. Heat up the same pan with the rest of the oil over medium-high heat, add tomatoes and cook them for 8 minutes stirring from time to time.
4. Return eggplant pieces to the pan and add a pinch of salt, black pepper, basil, mint and Tabasco sauce.
5. Stir, cook for 2 minutes more, divide between plates and serve.
6. Enjoy!

Nutritional value/serving:

calories 258, fat 25,6, fiber 5,1, carbs 9,5, protein 1.9

Eggplant Jam

Preparation time: 10 minutes

Cooking time: 1 hour

Servings: 6

Ingredients:

- 3 eggplants, sliced lengthwise
- 2 teaspoons sweet paprika
- 2 garlic cloves, minced
- A pinch of cinnamon, ground
- A pinch of sea salt
- 1 teaspoon cumin, ground
- A splash of hot sauce
- ¼ cup water
- 1 tablespoon parsley, chopped
- 2 tablespoons lemon juice

Directions:

1. Sprinkle some salt on eggplant slices and leave them aside for 10 minutes.
2. Pat dry eggplant, brush them with half of the oil, place on a lined baking sheet, place in the oven

at 375 degrees F, bake for 25 minutes flipping them halfway and leave them aside to cool down.
3. In a bowl, mix paprika with garlic, cinnamon, cumin, water and hot sauce and stir well.
4. Add baked eggplant pieces and mash them with a fork.
5. Heat up a pan with the rest of the oil over medium-low heat, add eggplant mix, stir and cook for 20 minutes.
6. Add lemon juice and parsley, stir, take off heat, divide into small bowls and serve.
7. Enjoy!

Nutritional value/serving:

calories 75, fat 0,7, fiber 10,1, carbs 17,2, protein 3

Artichokes and Tomatoes Dip

Preparation time: 10 minutes

Cooking time: 30 minutes

Servings: 4

Ingredients:

- 2 artichokes, cut in halves and trimmed
- Juice from 3 lemons
- 4 sun-dried tomatoes, chopped
- 1 garlic clove, minced
- 4 tablespoons olive oil
- A bunch of parsley, chopped
- A bunch of basil, chopped
- Black pepper to taste

Directions:

1. In a bowl, mix artichokes with lemon juice from 1 lemon, some black pepper and toss to coat.
2. Transfer to a large saucepan, add water to cover, bring to a boil over medium-high heat, cook for 30 minutes and drain.

3. In a food processor, mix the rest of the lemon juice with tomatoes, parsley, basil, garlic, black pepper and olive oil and blend well.
4. Divide artichokes between plates and top each with the tomatoes dip.
5. Enjoy!

Nutritional value/serving:

calories 193, fat 14,5, fiber 6,1, carbs 16,9, protein 4,1

Rhubarb and Strawberry Compote

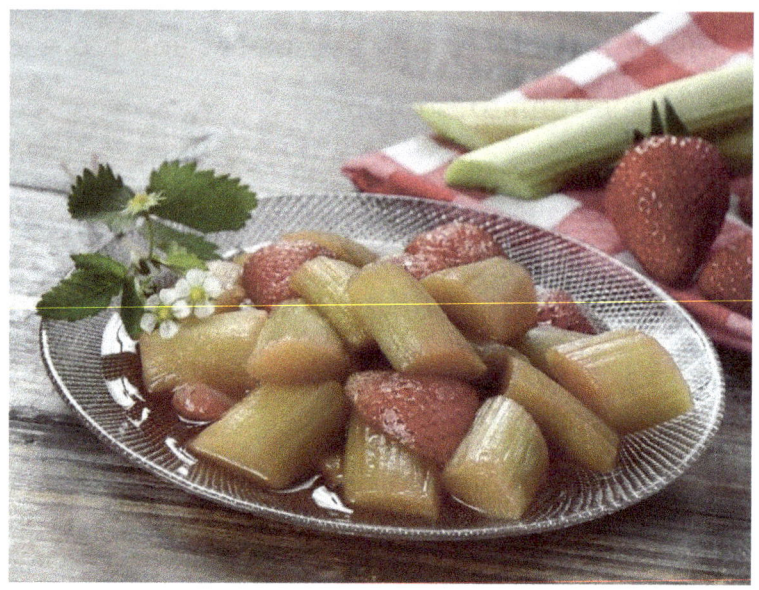

Preparation Time: 10 mins

Servings: 4

Ingredients:

- 2 lbs. rhubarb
- 1 lb. strawberries
- 3 tbsps. Date paste
- ½ c. water
- Fresh mint

Directions:

1. Peel the rhubarb using a paring knife and chop it up ½ inch pieces
2. Add the chopped up rhubarb to your pot alongside water
3. Lock up the lid and cook on HIGH pressure for 10 minutes
4. Stem and quarter your strawberries and keep them on the side
5. Add the strawberries and date paste, give it a nice stir
6. Lock up the lid and cook on HIGH pressure for 20 minutes
7. Release the pressure naturally and enjoy the compote!

Nutrition:

Calories: 41.1, Fat:2.1 g, Carbs:5.5 g, Protein:1.4 g, Sugars:12 g, Sodium:2.4 mg

Roasted Tomato Cream

Preparation time: 10 minutes

Cooking time: 1 hour

Servings: 8

Ingredients:

- 1 jalapeño pepper, chopped
- 4 garlic cloves, peeled and minced
- 1 onion, peeled and cut into wedges
- 2 pounds cherry tomatoes, cut in half
- ¼ cup olive oil
- ½ teaspoon dried oregano
- Salt and ground black pepper, to taste
- 4 cups chicken stock
- ¼ cup fresh basil, chopped
- ½ cup Parmesan cheese, grated

Directions:

1. Spread the tomatoes, and onion in a baking dish.
2. Add the garlic and chili pepper, season with salt, pepper, and oregano, and drizzle the oil.

3. Toss to coat and bake in the oven at 425 ºF for 30 minutes.
4. Take the tomato mixture out of the oven, transfer to a pot, add the stock, and heat everything up over medium-high heat.
5. Bring to a boil, cover the pot, reduce heat, and simmer for 20 minutes.
6. Blend using an immersion blender, add the salt and pepper to taste, and basil, stir, and ladle into soup bowls. Sprinkle with Parmesan cheese on top and serve.

Nutrition:

Calories - 140, Fat - 2, Fiber - 2, Carbs - 5, Protein - 8

Sweet Potato And Peanut Soup With Baby Spinach

Preparation Time: 5 Minutes

Cooking Time: 40 Minutes

Servings:4

Ingredients

- 1 medium onion, chopped
- 1 tablespoon olive oil
- 6 cups vegetable broth, homemade (see Light Vegetable Broth) or store-bought, or water
- 11/2 pounds sweet potatoes, peeled and cut into 1/2-inch dice
- 1/3 cup creamy peanut butter
- 1/4 teaspoon ground cayenne
- 1/8 teaspoon ground nutmeg
- Salt and freshly ground black pepper
- 4 cups fresh baby spinach

Directions

1. In a large soup pot, heat the oil over medium heat. Add the onion, cover, and cook until softened, about 5 minutes. Add the sweet potatoes and broth and cook, uncovered, until the potatoes are tender, about 30 minutes.
2. Ladle about a cup of hot broth into a small bowl. Add the peanut butter and stir until smooth. Stir the peanut butter mixture into the soup along with the cayenne, nutmeg, and salt and pepper to taste.
3. About 10 minutes before ready to serve, stir in the spinach, and serve.

Zoodle Bolognese

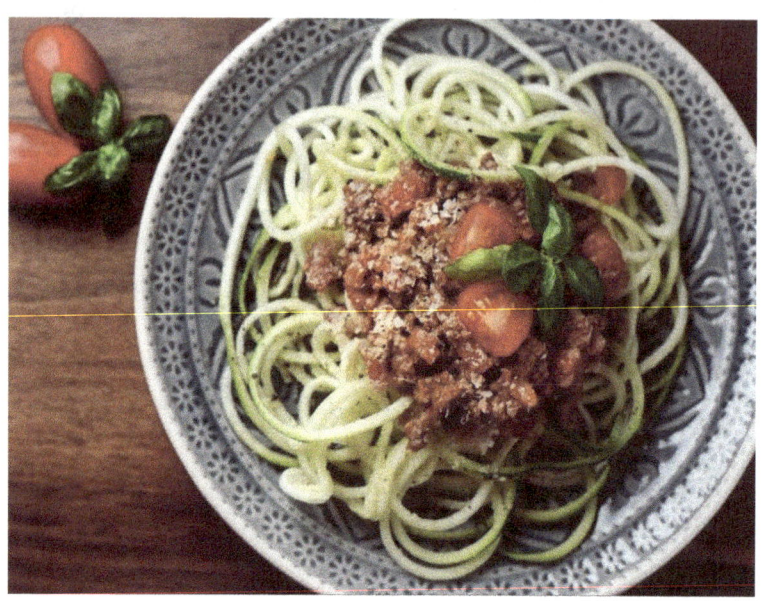

Preparation Time: 10minutes

Cooking Time: 35minutes

Serving: 4

Ingredients:

For the Bolognese sauce:

- 3 oz. olive oil
- 1 garlic clove, minced
- 1 white onion, chopped

- 3 oz. celery, chopped
- 3 cups crumbled tofu
- 2 tbsp tomato paste
- 1 ½ cups crushed tomatoes
- ¼ tsp black pepper
- 1 tsp salt
- 1 tbsp dried basil
- 1 tbsp Worcestershire sauce
- Water as needed

For the zoodles:

- 1 lb zucchinis
- 2 tbsp butter
- Salt and black pepper to taste

Directions:

1. Pour the olive oil into a saucepan and heat over medium heat. When no longer shimmering, add the onion, garlic, and celery. Sauté for 3 minutes or until the onions are soft and the carrots caramelized.
2. Pour in the tofu, tomato paste, tomatoes, salt, black pepper, basil, and Worcestershire sauce. Stir and cook for 15 minutes, or simmer for 30 minutes.

3. Mix in some water if the mixture is too thick and simmer further for 20 minutes.
4. While the sauce cooks, make the zoodles. Run the zucchini through a spiralizer to form noodles.
5. Melt the butter in a skillet over medium heat and toss the zoodles quickly in the butter, about 1 minute only.
6. Season with salt and black pepper.

Nutrition:

Calories: ,239 Total Fat:14.7g, Saturated Fat:8.1g, Total Carbs: 14g, Dietary Fiber:1g, Sugar:7 g, Protein: 13g, Sodium: 530mg

Keto Pasta with Mediterranean Tofu balls

Preparation Time: 90 minutes + overnight chilling

Serving size: 4

Ingredients:

For the keto pasta:

- 1 cup shredded mozzarella cheese
- 1 egg yolk

For the sauce:

- 3 tbsp olive oil
- 2 yellow onions, chopped
- 2 tbsp unsweetened tomato paste
- 6 garlic cloves, minced
- 2 large tomatoes, chopped
- ¼ tsp saffron powder
- 2 cinnamon sticks
- 4 ½ cups vegetable broth
- Salt and black pepper to taste

For the Mediterranean meatballs:

- 2 cups mushroom rinds
- 1 egg
- 1 lb tofu

- ¼ cup almond milk
- 6 garlic cloves, minced
- Salt and black pepper to taste
- ½ tsp coriander powder
- ¼ tsp nutmeg powder
- 1 tbsp smoked paprika
- 1 ½ tsp fresh ginger paste
- 1 tsp cumin powder
- ½ tsp cayenne pepper
- 1 ½ tsp turmeric powder
- ½ tsp cloves powder
- 4 tbsp chopped cilantro
- 4 tbsp chopped scallions
- 4 tbsp chopped parsley
- ¼ cup almond flour
- ¼ cup olive oil
- 1 cup crumbled cottage cheese for serving

Directions:

For the pasta:

1. Pour the cheese into a medium safe-microwave bowl and melt in the microwave for 35 minutes or until melted.

2. Remove the bowl and allow cooling for 1 minute only to warm the cheese but not cool completely. Mix in the egg yolk until well combined.
3. Lay parchment paper on a flat surface, pour the cheese mixture on top and cover with another parchment paper. Using a rolling pin, flatten the dough into 1/8-inch thickness.
4. Take off the parchment paper and cut the dough into spaghetti strands. Place in a bowl and refrigerate overnight.
5. When ready to cook, bring 2 cups of water to a boil in a medium saucepan and add the pasta.
6. Cook for 40 seconds to 1 minute and then drain through a colander. Run cold water over the pasta and set aside to cool.

For the Mediterranean tofu balls:

7. In a large pot, heat the olive oil and sauté the onions until softened, 3 minutes. Stir in the garlic and cook until fragrant, 30 seconds.
8. Stir in the tomato paste, tomatoes, saffron, and cinnamon sticks; cook for 2 minutes and then mix in the vegetable broth, salt, and black pepper. Simmer for 20 to 25 minutes while you

make the tofu balls.

9. In a large bowl, mix the mushroom rinds, tofu, egg, almond milk, garlic, salt, black pepper, coriander, nutmeg powder, paprika, ginger paste, cumin powder, cayenne pepper, turmeric powder, cloves powder, cilantro, parsley, 3 tablespoons of scallions, and almond flour. Form 1-inch meatballs from the mixture.
10. Heat the olive oil in a large skillet and fry the tofu balls in batches until brown on all sides, 10 minutes.
11. Put the tofu balls into the sauce, coat well with the sauce and continue cooking over low heat for 5 to 10 minutes.
12. Divide the pasta onto serving plates and spoon the tofu balls with sauce on top.
13. Garnish with the cottage cheese, remaining scallions and serve warm.

Nutrition:

Calories: 232, Total Fat:14.3g, Saturated Fat:5.4g, Total Carbs: 12g, Dietary Fiber:g4, Sugar:4 g, Protein:20 g, Sodium: 719mg

Spinach Salad With Orange-Dijon Dressing

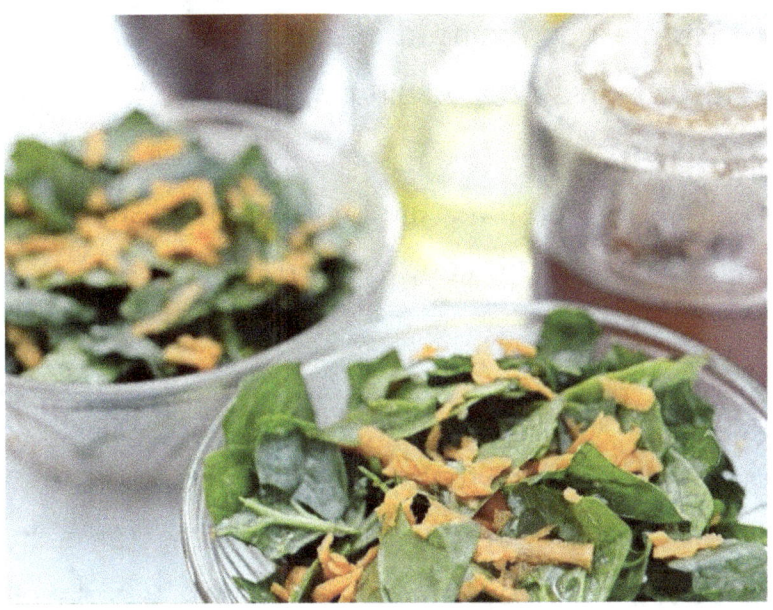

Preparation time: 10 minutes

cooking time: 0 minutes

servings: 4

Ingredients

- 2 tablespoons Dijon mustard
- 1/4 cup fresh orange juice
- 2 tablespoons olive oil

- 1 teaspoon agave nectar
- 2 tablespoons minced fresh parsley
- 1/2 teaspoon salt
- 1/4 teaspoon freshly ground black pepper
- 1 tablespoon minced green onions
- 5 cups fresh baby spinach, torn into bite-size pieces
- 1 navel orange, peeled and segmented
- 1/2 small red onion, sliced paper thin

Directions

1. In a blender or food processor combine the mustard, oil, orange juice, agave nectar, salt, pepper, parsley, and green onions. Blend well and set aside.
2. In a large bowl, combine the spinach, orange, and onion. Add the dressing, toss gently to combine, and serve.

Warm Lentil Salad with Red Wine Vinaigrette

Preparation time: 10 minutes

cooking time: 50 minutes

servings: 4

Ingredients

- 1 teaspoon olive oil plus ¼ cup, divided, or 1 tablespoon vegetable broth or water
- 1 carrot, diced
- 1 cup lentils
- 1 small onion, diced
- 1 garlic clove, minced
- 1 tablespoon dried basil
- 1 tablespoon dried oregano
- 1 tablespoon red wine or balsamic vinegar (optional)
- 2 cups water
- ¼ cup red wine vinegar or balsamic vinegar
- 1 teaspoon sea salt
- 2 cups chopped Swiss chard
- 2 cups torn red leaf lettuce
- 4 tablespoons Cheesy Sprinkle

Directions

1. Heat 1 teaspoon of the oil in a large pot on medium heat, then sauté the onion and garlic until they are translucent, about 5 minutes.
2. Add the carrot and sauté until it is slightly cooked, about 3 minutes.
3. Stir in the lentils, basil, and oregano, then add the wine or balsamic vinegar (if using).
4. Pour the water into the pot and turn the heat up to high to bring to a boil.
5. Turn the heat down to a simmer and let the lentils cook, uncovered, 20 to 30 minutes, until they are soft but not falling apart.
6. While the lentils are cooking, whisk together the red wine vinegar, olive oil, and salt in a small bowl and set aside.
7. Once the lentils have cooked, drain any excess liquid and stir in most of the red wine vinegar dressing. Set a little bit of dressing aside.
8. Add the Swiss chard to the pot and stir it into the lentils. Leave the heat on low and cook, stirring, for at least 10 minutes.

9. Toss the lettuce with the remaining dressing. Place some lettuce on a plate, and top with the lentil mixture.
10. Finish the plate off with a little Cheesy
11. Sprinkle and enjoy.

Nutrition

Calories: 387; Total fat: 17g; Carbs: 42g; Fiber: 19g; Protein: 18g

Tabbouleh Salad

Preparation time: 15 minutes

cooking time: 10 minutes

servings: 4

Ingredients

- 1 cup whole-wheat couscous
- 1 cup boiling water
- 1 garlic clove, pressed
- Zest and juice of 1 lemon
- Pinch sea salt
- 1 tablespoon olive oil, or flaxseed oil (optional)
- ½ cucumber, diced small
- 1 tomato, diced small
- 1 cup fresh parsley, chopped
- ¼ cup fresh mint, finely chopped
- 2 scallions, finely chopped
- 4 tablespoons sunflower seeds (optional)

Directions

1. Put the couscous in a medium bowl, and cover with boiling water until all the grains are submerged. Cover the bowl with a plate or wrap. Set aside.
2. Put the lemon zest and juice in a large salad bowl, then stir in the garlic, salt, and the olive oil (if using).
3. Put the cucumber, tomato, parsley, mint, and scallions in the bowl, and toss them to coat with the dressing. Take the plate off the couscous and fluff with a fork.
4. Add the cooked couscous to the vegetables, and toss to combine.
5. Serve topped with the sunflower seeds (if using).

Nutrition

Calories: 304; Total fat: 11g; Carbs: 44g; Fiber: 6g; Protein: 10g

Yellow Mung Bean Salad With Broccoli And Mango

Preparation Time: 5 Minutes

Cooking Time: 20 Minutes

Servings:4

Ingredients

- 1/2 cup yellow mung beans, picked over, rinsed, and drained
- 1 jalapeño or other hot green chile, seeded and minced
- 3 cups small broccoli florets, blanched
- 1 ripe mango, peeled, pitted, and chopped
- 1 small red bell pepper, chopped
- 2 tablespoons chopped fresh cilantro
- 1 teaspoon grated fresh ginger
- 2 tablespoons fresh lemon juice
- 3 tablespoons grapeseed oil
- 1/3 cup unsalted roasted cashews for garnish

Directions

1. In a saucepan of boiling salted water, cook the mung beans until just tender, 18 to 20 minutes. Drain and run under cold water to cool.
2. Transfer the beans to a large bowl. Add the broccoli, mango, bell pepper, chile, and cilantro. Set aside.
3. In a small bowl, combine the ginger, lemon juice, oil. Stir to mix well, then pour the dressing over the vegetables and toss to combine.
4. Sprinkle with cashews and serve.

Baked Onion Rings

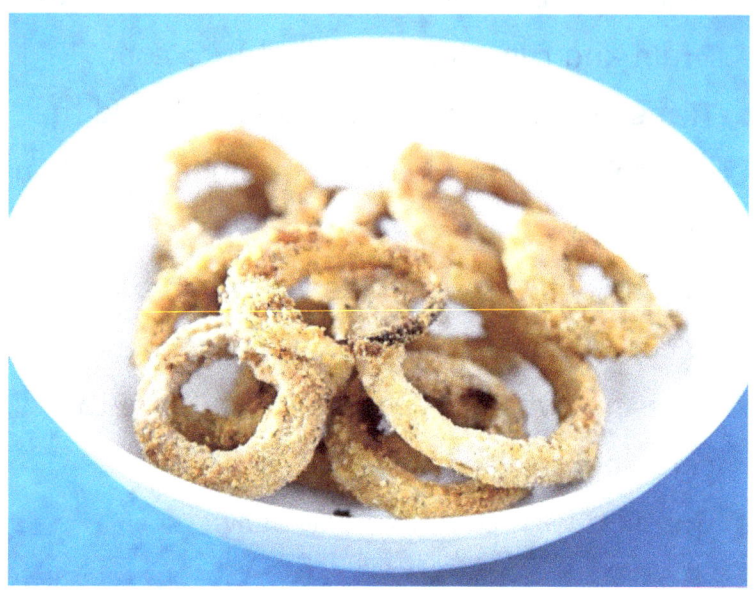

Preparation Time: 5 minutes

Cooking Time: 25 minutes

Servings: 4

Ingredients:

- 2 eggs, organic
- ½ teaspoon pepper
- ½ teaspoon garlic powder
- ½ teaspoon salt

- 2 tablespoons thyme, sliced
- 1 ½ cups almond flour
- 2 large sweet onions, cut into rings

Directions:

1. Preheat your oven to 400° fahrenheit.
2. In a mixing bowl, combine garlic powder, almond flour, thyme, garlic powder, and salt.
3. Take another bowl, add eggs and whisk.
4. Dip the onion ring in egg mixture then coat with flour mixture.
5. Place the coated onion rings in a baking dish.
6. Bake in preheated oven for 25 minutes.
7. Serve immediately and enjoy!

Nutrition:

Calories: 130 Carbohydrates: 10.7 G Fat: 7.4 G
Sugar: 3.5 G Cholesterol: 82 Mg Protein: 6.1 G

Corn Cream Soup

Preparation time: 10 minutes

Cooking time: 8 hours and 10 minutes

Servings: 6

Ingredients:

- 1 yellow onion, chopped
- 2 tablespoons olive oil
- 1 red bell pepper, chopped
- 3 cups gold potatoes, chopped
- 4 cups veggie stock
- 4 cups corn kernels
- ½ teaspoon smoked paprika
- 1 teaspoon cumin, ground
- Salt and black pepper to the taste
- 1 cup almond milk
- 2 scallions, chopped

Directions:

1. Heat up a pan with the oil over medium high heat, add onion, stir and cook for 5-6 minutes.

2. Transfer this to your slow cooker, add bell pepper, potatoes, 3 cups corn, stock, paprika, cumin, salt and pepper, stir, cover and cook on Low for 7 hours and 30 minutes.
3. Blend soup using an immersion blender, add almond milk and blend again.
4. Add the rest of the corn, cover pot and cook on Low for 30 minutes more.
5. Ladle soup into bowls, sprinkle scallions on top and serve.
6. Enjoy!

Nutrition:

calories 312, fat 4, fiber 6, carbs 12, protein 4

Corn And Cabbage Soup

Preparation time: 10 minutes

Cooking time: 7 hours

Servings: 4

Ingredients:

- 1 small yellow onion, chopped
- 1 tablespoon olive oil
- 2 garlic cloves, minced
- 1 and ½ cups mushrooms, sliced
- 2 cups corn kernels
- 4 cups red cabbage, chopped
- 3 teaspoons ginger, grated
- A pinch of salt and black pepper
- 4 cups water
- 1 tablespoon nutritional yeast
- 1 teaspoon sesame oil
- 2 teaspoons tomato paste
- 1 teaspoon coconut aminos
- 1 teaspoon sriracha sauce

Directions:

1. In your slow cooker, mix olive oil with onion, garlic, mushrooms, ginger, salt, pepper, corn, cabbage, water, yeast and tomato paste, stir, cover and cook on Low for 7 hours.
2. Add sriracha sauce and aminos, stir, leave soup aside for a few minutes, ladle into bowls, drizzle sesame oil all over and serve.
3. Enjoy!

Nutrition:

calories 300, fat 4, fiber 4, carbs 10, protein 4

Okra Soup

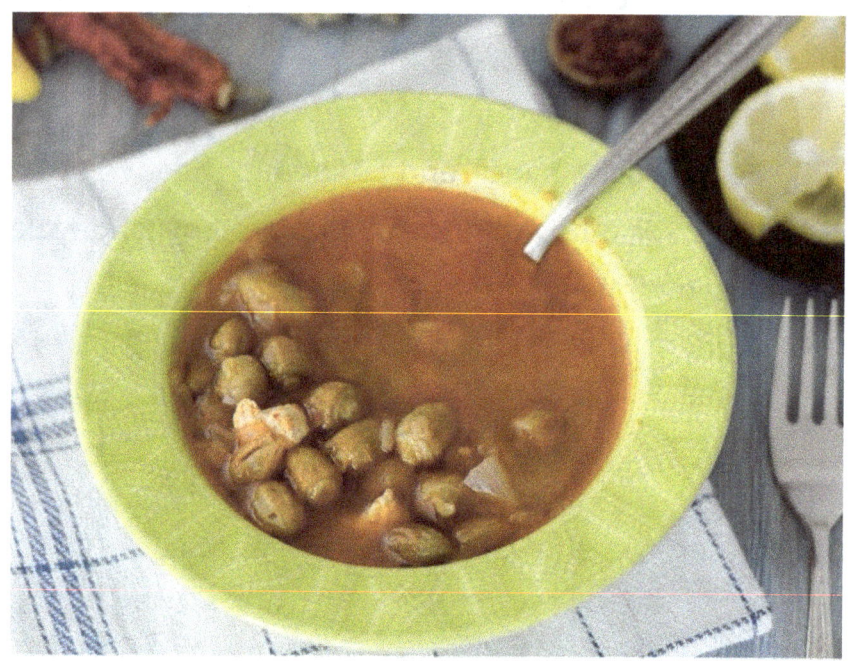

Preparation time: 10 minutes

Cooking time: 5 hours

Servings: 6

Ingredients:

- 1 small yellow onion, chopped
- 1 green bell pepper, chopped
- 3 cups veggie stock

- 3 garlic cloves, minced
- 16 ounces okra, sliced
- 29 ounces canned tomatoes, crushed
- 2 cup corn
- 1 and ½ teaspoon smoked paprika
- 1 teaspoon marjoram, dried
- 1 teaspoon thyme, dried
- 1 teaspoon oregano, dried
- Salt and black pepper to the taste

Directions:

1. In your slow cooker, mix bell pepper with onion, stock, garlic, okra, corn, tomatoes, smoked paprika, marjoram, thyme, oregano, salt and pepper, stir, cover and cook on High for 5 hours.
2. Ladle into bowls and serve.
3. Enjoy!

Nutrition:

calories 243, fat 4, fiber 6, carbs 10, protein 3

Baby Carrots And Coconut Soup

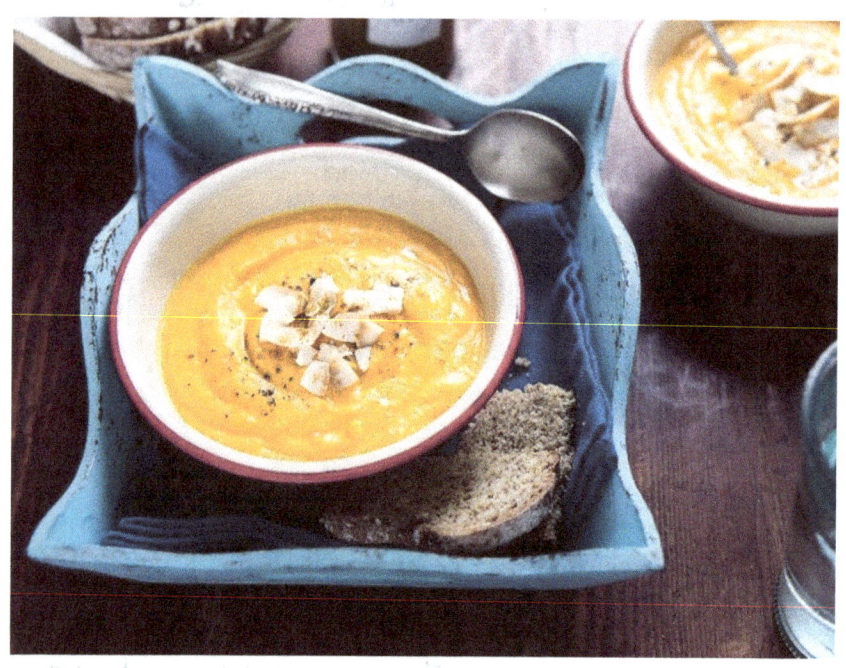

Preparation time: 10 minutes

Cooking time: 7 hours

Servings: 6

Ingredients:

- 1 yellow onion, chopped
- 1 sweet potato, cubed
- 2 pounds baby carrots, peeled

- 2 teaspoons ginger paste
- 4 cups veggie stock
- 2 teaspoons curry powder
- Salt and black pepper to the taste
- 14 ounces coconut milk

Directions:

1. In your slow cooker, mix sweet potato with baby carrots, ginger paste, onion, stock, curry powder, salt and pepper, stir, cover and cook on High for 7 hours.
2. Add coconut milk, blend soup using an immersion blender, divide soup into bowls and serve.
3. Enjoy!

Nutrition:

calories 100, fat 2, fiber 4, carbs 18, protein 3

Nut Free Nacho Dip (vegan)

Preparation time: 15 minutes

Cooking time: 0 minute

Servings: 8

Ingredients:

- 1 large eggplant (peeled and cubed)
- 2 medium Hass avocados (peeled, pitted, and halved)
- ¼ cup MCT oil
- 2 tsp. nutritional yeast
- 1 jalapeno pepper
- 1 red onion (diced)
- 1 garlic clove (halved)
- ¼ cup fresh cilantro (chopped)
- 1 tsp. cumin seeds
- 1 tbsp. paprika powder
- 1 tsp. dried oregano
- ½ tsp. Himalayan salt

Directions:

1. Slice the jalapeno in half lengthwise; remove the seeds, stem, and placenta, and discard.
2. Put the jalapeno and all other ingredients in a food processor or blender.
3. Mix everything into a smooth mixture. Use a spatula to scrape down the sides of the blender to make sure everything gets mixed evenly.
4. Transfer the dip to an airtight container.
5. Serve, share, and enjoy!
6. Alternatively, store the cheese in an airtight container in the fridge and consume within 2 days.

Nutrition:

Calories: 135kcal, Net Carbs: 3.5g, Fat: 12.3g, Protein: 1.8g, Fiber: 5.4g, Sugar: 2.7g

Black Olive & Thyme Cheese Spread (vegan)

Preparation time: 25 minutes

Cooking time: 15 minutes

Servings: 16

Ingredients:

- 1 cup macadamia nuts (unsalted)
- 1 cup pine nuts
- 1 tsp. thyme (finely chopped)
- 1 tsp. rosemary (finely chopped)
- 2 tsp. nutritional yeast
- 1 tsp. Himalayan salt
- 10 black olives (pitted, finely chopped)

Directions:

1. Preheat the oven to 350°F / 175°C, and line a baking sheet with parchment paper.
2. Put the nuts on a baking sheet, and spread them out so they can roast evenly. Transfer the baking sheet to the oven and roast the nuts for about 8 minutes, until slightly browned.

3. Take the nuts out of the oven and set aside for about 4 minutes, allowing them to cool down.
4. Add all ingredients to a blender and process until everything combines into a smooth mixture. Use a spatula to scrape down the sides of the blender container in between blending to make sure everything gets mixed evenly.
5. Serve, share, and enjoy!
6. Alternatively, store the cheese in an airtight container in the fridge and consume within 6 days. Store for a maximum of 60 days in the freezer and thaw at room temperature.

Nutrition:

Calories: 118kcal, Net Carbs: 0.7g, Fat: 11.9g, Protein: 2g, Fiber: 1.4g, Sugar: 0.7g

Curry with Bok Choy

Preparation Time: 15 minutes

Cooking Time: 15 minutes

Servings: 3

Ingredients:

- 2 tablespoons extra virgin coconut oil or olive oil
- 1 small onion, peeled, finely diced
- 2 cloves garlic, peeled, finely chopped
- 1 tablespoon curry powder
- ½ teaspoon ground turmeric
- 1 tablespoon fresh grated ginger
- ½ teaspoon ground fenugreek
- 14 oz. unsweetened coconut milk
- 2 bok choy, washed, feet removed, roughly chopped (14 oz.)
- ½ cup vegetable stock

For serving:

- Lemon juice
- Fresh coriander
- Chili flake

Directions:

1. Place a large skillet over medium heat and add oil. Once the oil is heated, add onions and garlic and cook 1-2 minutes or until golden brown, taking care not to burn them.
2. Add curry powder, grated ginger, turmeric and fenugreek. Stir fry 30 seconds to 1 minute until fragrant.
3. Stir in bok choy then cover, turn the heat down to medium-low, and cook 3-4 minutes.
4. Increase the heat to medium-high, uncover and cook 3 - 4 minutes to evaporate the vegetable juice slightly.
5. Pour in coconut milk and vegetable stock; cook an additional 10 minutes until a thick liquid reduces.
6. Place curry in a serving bowl. Drizzle with lemon juice. Sprinkle with freshly chopped coriander and chili flakes.

Nutrition:

Calories: 200, Total Fats: 15.3g, Carbohydrates: 13.4g, Fiber: 4.8g, Protein: 4.7g, Sugar: 5.2

Capers Dip

Preparation time: 10 minutes

Cooking time: 20 minutes

Servings: 4

Ingredients:

- 2 tablespoons olive oil
- 4 scallions, chopped
- 2 tablespoons capers, drained
- 1 teaspoon rosemary, dried
- 1 cup coconut cream
- 2 tablespoons pine nuts
- 1 bunch basil, chopped

Directions:

1. Heat up a pan with the oil over medium heat, add the scallions and the capers and sauté for 5 minutes.
2. Add the cream and the other ingredients, stir, cook over medium heat for 15 minutes more, blend using an immersion blender, divide into bowls and serve.

Nutrition:

calories 127, fat 3, fiber 3, carbs 6, protein 7

Apple Crumble

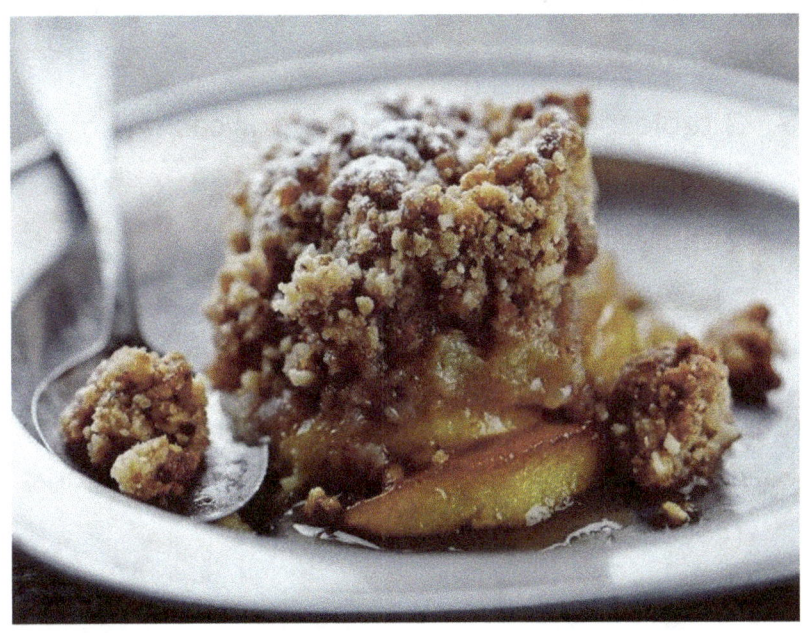

Preparation time: 20 minutes

cooking time: 25 minutes

servings: 6

Ingredients

For the filling

- 4 to 5 apples, cored and chopped (about 6 cups)
- ½ cup unsweetened applesauce, or ¼ cup water
- 2 to 3 tablespoons unrefined sugar (coconut,

date, sucanat, maple syrup)
- 1 teaspoon ground cinnamon
- Pinch sea salt

For the crumble

- 2 tablespoons almond butter, or cashew or sunflower seed butter
- 2 tablespoons maple syrup
- 1½ cups rolled oats
- ½ cup walnuts, finely chopped
- ½ teaspoon ground cinnamon
- 2 to 3 tablespoons unrefined granular sugar (coconut, date, sucanat)

Directions

1. Preheat the oven to 350 °F. Put the apples and applesauce in an 8-inch-square baking dish, and sprinkle with the sugar, cinnamon, and salt. Toss to combine.
2. In a medium bowl, mix together the nut butter and maple syrup until smooth and creamy.
3. Add the oats, walnuts, cinnamon, and sugar and stir to coat, using your hands if necessary. (If you have a small food processor, pulse the oats and walnuts together before adding them to the

mix.
4. Sprinkle the topping over the apples, and put the dish in the oven.
5. Bake for 20 to 25 minutes, or until the fruit is soft and the topping is lightly browned.

Nutrition

Calories: 356; Total fat: 17g; Carbs: 49g; Fiber: 7g; Protein: 7g

Peach-Mango Crumble (Pressure cooker)

Preparation time: 10 minutes

Servings: 4-6

Ingredients

- 3 cups chopped fresh or frozen peaches
- 3 cups chopped fresh or frozen mangos
- ½ cup shredded coconut, sweetened or unsweetened
- 4 tablespoons unrefined sugar or pure maple syrup, divided
- 1 cup gluten-free rolled oats
- 2 tablespoons coconut oil or vegan margarine

Directions

1. In a 6- to 7-inch round baking dish, toss together the peaches, mangos, and 2 tablespoons of sugar. In a food processor, combine the oats, coconut, coconut oil, and remaining 2 tablespoons of sugar. Pulse until combined. (If you use maple syrup, you'll need less coconut oil. Start with just the syrup and

add oil if the mixture isn't sticking together. Sprinkle the oat mixture over the fruit mixture.
2. Cover the dish with aluminum foil. Put a trivet in the bottom of your electric pressure cooker's cooking pot and pour in a cup or two of water. Using a foil sling or silicone helper handles, lower the pan onto the trivet.
3. High pressure for 6 minutes. Close and lock the lid and ensure the pressure valve is sealed, then select High Pressure and set the time for 6 minutes.
4. Pressure Release. Once the cook time is complete, quick release the pressure, being careful not to get your fingers or face near the steam release. Once all the pressure has released, carefully unlock and remove the lid.
5. Let cool for a few minutes before carefully lifting out the dish with oven mitts or tongs. Scoop out portions to serve.

Nutrition

Calories: 321; Total fat: 18g; Protein: 4g; Sodium: 2mg; Fiber: 7g

Coconut and Almond Truffles

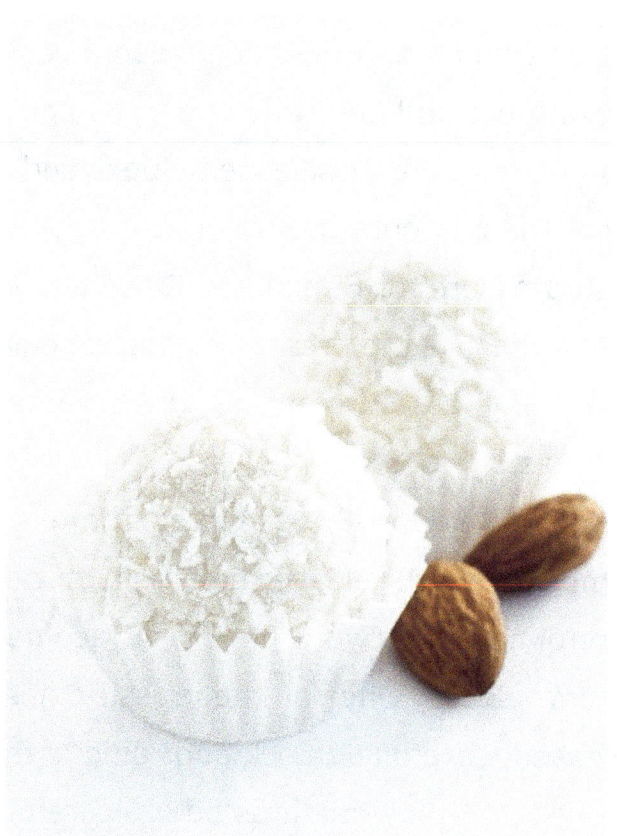

Preparation time: 15 minutes

cooking time: 0 minutes

servings: 8 truffles

Ingredients

- 1 cup pitted dates
- 1 cup almonds
- ½ cup sweetened cocoa powder, plus extra for coating
- 1 teaspoon vanilla extract
- ½ cup unsweetened shredded coconut
- ¼ cup pure maple syrup
- 1 teaspoon almond extract
- ¼ teaspoon sea salt

Directions

1. In the bowl of a food processor, combine all the ingredients and process until smooth. Chill the mixture for about 1 hour.
2. Roll the mixture into balls and then roll the balls in cocoa powder to coat.
3. Serve immediately or keep chilled until ready to serve.

Avocado and Pineapple Bowls

Preparation time: 10 minutes

Cooking time: 0 minutes

Servings: 4

Ingredients:

- 2 tablespoons avocado oil
- 1 cup pineapple, peeled and cubed
- 2 avocados, peeled, pitted and cubed
- Juice of 1 lime
- 2 tablespoons stevia

Directions:

1. In a bowl, combine the pineapple with the avocados and the other ingredients, toss, and serve cold.

Nutrition:

calories 312, fat 29.5, fiber 3.3, carbs 16.7, protein 5

Mint Cookies

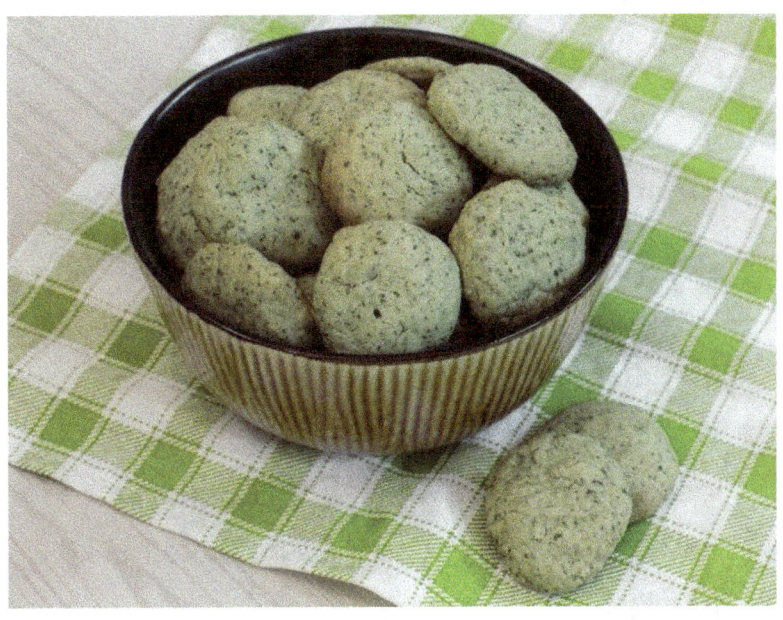

Preparation time: 10 minutes

Cooking time: 20 minutes

Servings: 6

Ingredients:

- 2 cups coconut flour
- 3 tablespoons flaxseed mixed with 4 tablespoons water
- ½ cup coconut oil, melted

- ½ cup coconut cream
- 3 tablespoons stevia
- 2 teaspoons mint, dried
- 2 teaspoons baking soda

Directions:

1. In a bowl, mix the coconut flour with the flaxseed, coconut cream and the other ingredients, and whisk really well.
2. Shape balls out of this mix, place them on a lined baking sheet, flatten them, introduce in the oven at 370 degrees F and bake for 20 minutes.
3. Serve the cookies cold.

Nutrition:

calories 190, fat 7.32, fiber 2.2, carbs 4, protein 3

Sweet Zucchini Buns

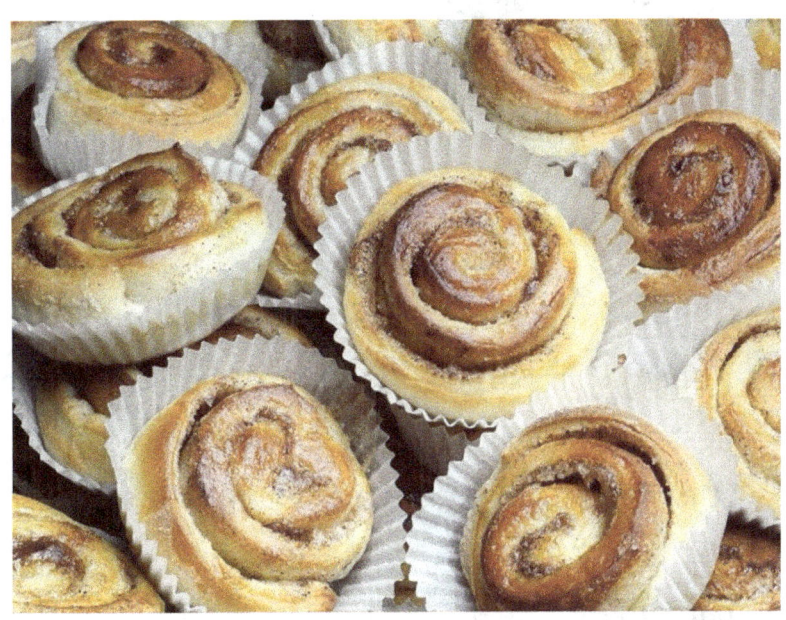

Preparation time: 10 minutes

Cooking time: 30 minutes

Servings: 8

Ingredients:

- 1 cup almond flour
- 1 cup zucchinis, grated
- 1/3 cup coconut flesh, unsweetened and shredded

- 1 cup coconut cream
- 2 tablespoons stevia
- 1 teaspoon baking soda
- ½ teaspoon cinnamon powder
- 3 tablespoons flaxseed mixed with 4 tablespoons water

Directions:

1. In a bowl, mix the almond flour with the coconut flesh, the zucchinis and the other ingredients, stir well until you obtain a dough, shape 8 buns and arrange them on a baking sheet lined with parchment paper.
2. Introduce in the oven at 350 degrees and bake for 30 minutes.
3. Serve these sweet buns warm.

Nutrition:

calories 169, fat 15.3, fiber 3.9, carbs 6.4, protein 3.2

Peppermint Patty Cocoa

Preparation Time: 15 Minutes

Servings: 4

Ingredients:

- 4 cups almond milk
- 3 ounces semisweet chocolate chips
- 1/4 cup sugar
- 1 teaspoon cocoa powder
- 1 teaspoon vanilla extract
- 1 tablespoon agave nectar
- 1 teaspoon peppermint extract

Directions:

1. Combine all the ingredients in the Cooker. Seal the lid and cook on high 4 minutes, then let the pressure release naturally.
2. Serve garnished with a sprig of mint or topped with vegan marshmallows!

Maple & Rum Apples.

Preparation Time: 25 Minutes

Servings: 6

Ingredients:

- 6 Granny Smith apples, washed
- ½ cup pure maple syrup
- ¼ cup golden raisins
- ½ cup apple juice
- ⅓ cup packed light brown sugar
- ¼ cup dark rum or spiced rum
- ¼ cup old-fashioned rolled oats
- ¼ cup macadamia nut pieces
- 1 teaspoon ground cinnamon
- ½ teaspoon ground nutmeg
- Juice of 1 lemon

Directions:

1. Core the apples most of the way down, leaving a little base so the stuffing stays put.
2. Stand your apples upright in your Cooker. Do not pile them on top of each other! You may

need to do two batches.
3. In a bowl combine the oats, sugar, raisins, nuts, and half the nutmeg, half the cinnamon.
4. Stuff each apple with the mix.
5. In another bowl combine the remaining nutmeg and cinnamon, the maple syrup, and the rum.
6. Pour the glaze over the apples.
7. Seal and cook on Stew for 20 minutes.
8. Depressurize naturally.

Zucchini bread

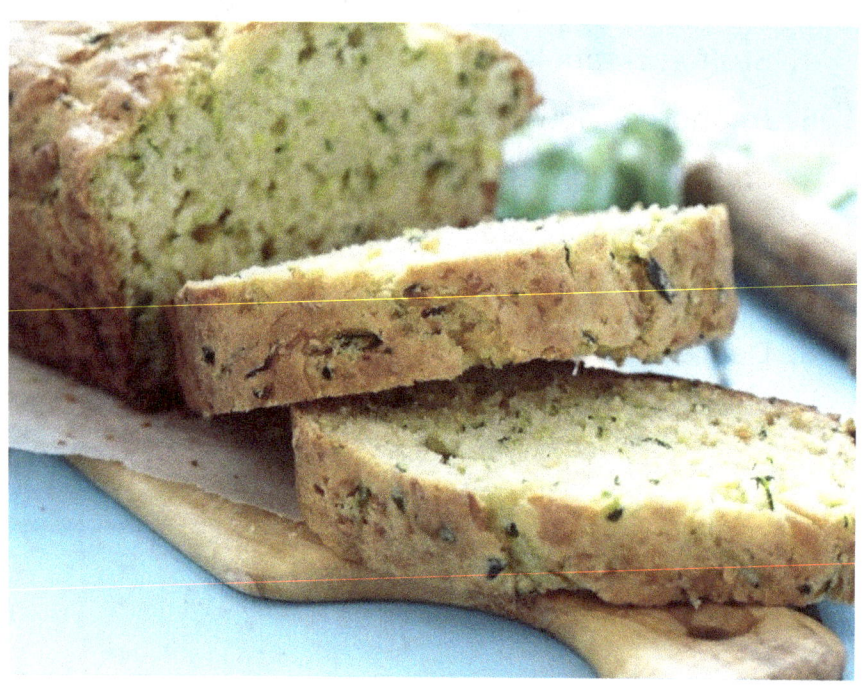

Preparation Time: 20 minutes

Cooking Time: 50 minutes

Servings: 12

Ingredients:

For the Loaf:

- 2 cups almond flour
- 2 teaspoons baking powder

- ½ teaspoon xanthan gum
- ¼ teaspoon salt
- ½ cup coconut oil, melted
- ¾ cup Swerve granular
- 3 large eggs
- 1 teaspoon vanilla extract
- 2 tablespoons fresh lemon juice
- 1 tablespoon lemon zest
- 1 cup zucchini shredded, drained

For the Glaze:

- ⅓ cup Swerve confectioners
- 4 tablespoons lemon juice

Directions:

1. Preheat oven to 325 °F. Cover the loaf pan with parchment paper.
2. Combine flour, salt, baking powder, and xanthan gum in a bowl. Mix well.
3. In a separate medium bowl, whisk together oil, Swerve granular, eggs, vanilla, and lemon juice.
4. Add the wet ingredients to the dry ingredients and mix until just combined.
5. Fold the zucchini and lemon zest into the batter.

6. Pour the batter into the prepared loaf pan and bake until a toothpick inserted into the middle comes out clean, about 50 minutes. If you find your zucchini bread is browning too quickly, you can cover the pan with foil.
7. Remove from the oven and let the bread cool in the pan for 10 minutes. Carefully remove the bread from the pan and cool completely on a wire rack.
8. Whisk together Swerve confectioners and lemon juice. Drizzle loaf with glaze.
9. Slice and serve.

Nutrition:

Calories: 143, Total Fats: 13g, Carbohydrates: 2g, Fiber: 1g, Protein: 2g

Fat-Rich Protein Espresso (vegan)

Preparation Time: 5 minutes

Cooking Time: 0 minute

Servings: 1

Ingredients:

- 1 cup espresso (freshly brewed)
- 2 tbsp. coconut butter (or alternatively, use coconut oil)
- 1 scoop organic soy protein (chocolate flavor)
- 4 ice cubes or ½ cup boiled water
- ½ vanilla stick
- 2 tbsp. coconut cream
- Optional: 1 tbsp. cacao powder
- Optional: ½ tsp. cinnamon

Directions:

1. Make sure to use fresh, hot espresso.
2. Add all the listed ingredients to a heat-safe blender, including the ice or boiled water and optional ingredients (if desired). Use ice to make iced espresso, or hot water for a warm treat.

3. Blend the ingredients for 1 minute and transfer to a large coffee cup.
4. Top the coffee with the coconut cream, stir, serve and enjoy!
5. Alternatively, store the smoothie in an airtight container or a mason jar, keep it in the fridge, and consume within 3 days. Store for a maximum of 30 days in the freezer and thaw at room temperature.

Nutrition:

Calories: 441kcal, Net Carbs: 5.6g, Fat: 34.8g, Protein: 25.4g, Fiber: 6.9g, Sugar: 2.8g

NOTE

www.ingramcontent.com/pod-product-compliance
Lightning Source LLC
Chambersburg PA
CBHW070101120526
44589CB00033B/1458